Vegan Diet

Vegan Clean Eating Diet Recipes: Healthy, Easy Prep Anti - Inflammation Recipes

(Easy Vegetarian Recipes And 21 Day Meal Plan for Guaranteed Weight Loss)

Daryl Morris

Published by Robert Satterfield Publishing House

© **Daryl Morris**

All Rights Reserved

Vegan Diet Cookbook: Vegan Clean Eating Diet Recipes: Healthy, Easy Prep Anti - Inflammation Recipes (Easy Vegetarian Recipes And 21 Day Meal Plan for Guaranteed Weight Loss)

ISBN 978-1-989787-17-5

All rights reserved. No part of this guide may be reproduced in any form without permission in writing from the publisher except in the case of brief quotations embodied in critical articles or reviews.

Legal & Disclaimer

The information contained in this book is not designed to replace or take the place of any form of medicine or professional medical advice. The information in this book has been provided for educational and entertainment purposes only.

The information contained in this book has been compiled from sources deemed reliable, and it is accurate to the best of the Author's knowledge; however, the Author cannot guarantee its accuracy and validity and cannot be held liable for any errors or omissions. Changes are periodically made to this book. You must consult your doctor or get professional medical advice before using any of the suggested remedies, techniques, or information in this book.

TABLE OF CONTENT

Part 1 1

Introduction 2

Chapter 1: T Benefits Of Living A Vegan Lifestyle 3

Chapter 2: Ten Tips For New Vegans 7

Chapter 3: Five Ways To Make Your Vegan Meals Taste Amazing 14

Vegan Breakfast Recipes 19

Lemon Scones Vegan Style 20

Blueberry And Cornmeal Pancakes 21

Vegan Style Crepes 23

Breakfast Style Raisin And Rice Pudding 25

Breakfast Strawberry And Oatmeal Smoothie 26

Vegan Style Apple And Carrot Breakfast Muffins 27

Healthy Banana And Kale Smoothie 29

Classic Oat Bran Cereal 31

Vegan Lunch Recipes 32

Spicy Lentil Wraps 32

Delicious Quinoa Salad With Fresh Avocado And Dill 35

Vegan Style Mac And Cheese 37

Hearty Zucchini And Red Pepper Stew 39

Vegan Style Black Bean Quesadillas 41

- Scrambled Up Tofu 43
- Asian Style Lettuce Wraps 44
- Classic Chickpea Curry 46
- Vegan Dinner Recipes... 47
- Vegan Style Fajitas.. 47
- Vegan Style Spicy Potato Curry 49
- Delicious Avocado Tacos 52
- Traditional Vegan Quinoa Chard Pilaf 53
- Vegan Style Shepherd's Pie 54
- Mediterranean Zucchini 57
- Delicious Tomato Pasta 59
- Teriyaki Style Tofu With Pineapple 60
- Vegan Desserts 62
- Vegan Style Cupcakes 62
- Mouthwatering Tofu Pumpkin Pie 64
- Vegan Style Brownies 66
- Strawberries Mixed With Balsamic Vinegar 67
- Vegan Style Chocolate Pudding............................ 68
- Delicious Vegan Style Chocolate Cake................ 69
- Banana Flavored Cookies 70
- Basic Vanilla Cake 72
- Conclusion 74

- Part 2 76
- Sweet Potato Chickpea-Less Hummus Vegan Bowl 77
- Quinoa Cauliflower With Almond Sauce Bowl 80
- Superfood Quinoa Bowl 84
- Burrito-Added Cauliflower Rice Bowl.................................. 86
- Marinated Tofu Brown Rice Bowl... 89
- Chickpeas And Roasted Cauliflower Bowl With Lemon-Dijon Dressing... 92
- Falafel Roasted Chickpeas Entree 94
- Cranberry Vegan Salad Sandwich.. 97
- Roasty Soba Entrée 99
- Peas Shallots Burmese Fried Rice...................................... 101
- Cauliflower With Orange Sauce Entrée............................. 103
- About The Author... 106

Part 1

Introduction

For those who claim that being a Vegan is not only a lifestyle choice, but also a philosophy, they couldn't be more correct. If you are reading this cookbook, then chances are that you are a Vegan and as such you know the reasons as to why you became a Vegan in the first place.

Regardless of the reason you decided to become a vegan, you have started to live a lifestyle that will leave you feeling better and healthier than you ever felt before. It is no secret that you will benefit greatly from this diet and that you will live a much healthier life in the long run.

In this book you will find a variety of healthy and delicious Vegan recipes, all designed to help you live the healthiest lifestyle that you could possibly live. All of the recipes that you will find in this book are incredibly easy to make and will help you to make the most out of your Vegan diet.

Chapter 1: T Benefits of Living A Vegan Lifestyle

There are many reasons why people decide to go Vegan and each person has their own story to tell about their journey to Veganism. However, there is one thing that every Vegan shares in common and that is the awesome benefits they are reaping while on this diet together.

There are three primary reasons why many people choose to adopt a Vegan lifestyle, but they are in no way the only reasons. These three popular reasons include:

1. Wanting To Be Fair To Animals

Being on a Vegan diet means that a person will not consume any food item that is of animal origin and they will not use any products that originate from animals. This means that Vegan will not touch dairy or egg products, even though these items do not kill the animal in the process or even use leather if it comes from an animal.

Many Vegans and people believe that animals should be able to exist on our planet, without interference from humans. Because of this reasoning many Vegans would rather sacrifice delicious meats and products for the good of animals and are happy doing so.

2. Wanting To Help The Environment

It is no secret that our planet has taken years and years of abuse from humans. Whether it is from global warming or harming our ozone layer, we are slowly destroying our planet. Because of this many Vegans believe that animal farming is something that is completely inefficient. The reason they believe this is because animal feed productions takes up a lot of land, water and resources that could be better spent helping our planet rather than destroying one of its inhabitants.

One of the most popular beliefs of Vegans who share this point of view is that investing in these livestock farms is the primary reason most of the earth's topsoil is eroding. Without this important topsoil, we are not able to cultivate our crops. In all reality the entire earth's population could be fed on the land we currently have if only the entire population became Vegan.

3. Want To Improve Their Overall Health

It is no secret that meat and fat has had a proven track record of doing more harm to a person's body then good. Consuming animal fats and animal protein have been linked to the development of diabetes, heart disease, cancer, high blood pressure, arthritis and various other medical ailments. There have also been numerous studies conducted that have shown meat eaters are also most likely to die prematurely then those that consume only plant based items.

Why is this? It is simply because our bodies are not designed to digest cow's milk, animal meat and the numerous types of animal fat out there. There have been numerous studies down that have found that people who solely consume plant based diets are either able to minimize the risk of developing chronic illnesses or they are able to live a much longer and healthy life in the long run.

What Are The Risks?

Surprisingly there is only one risk to becoming Vegan and it is one that many Vegans are not aware of prior to starting their new lifestyle. One of the things that Vegans will have to be wary of is Vitamin B12 Deficiency. The reason why this is so common among Vegans is because our bodies cannot use the plant form of this vitamin and so we cannot get an adequate amount into our bodies on a daily basis. Since this is very common among Vegans today it is extremely important that Vegans use a Vitamin B12 supplement on a daily basis to prevent this from happening.

Chapter 2: Ten Tips For New Vegans

Starting something new can be both exciting and very scary all at the same time. However, there are a few things that many Vegans should all know and consider before fully committing to this lifestyle and in this chapter you will learn for yourself what helpful tips you will need in order to be a successful Vegan.

1. Have An Open Mind

There is no way faster to failure than having a certain way of negative thinking and attitude towards your new diet. This cannot be any truer for the Vegan diet and lifestyle and this is something that is not going to be easy for many people to commit to. Try to think very positive about this endeavor. If you go into it thinking that you are just punishing yourself and that it will not last forever, trust me it won't. That is the kind of thing that you want to avoid.

2. If Cooking At Home, Make Sure You Give Yourself Plenty of Time To Do So

There is nothing worse than making a fresh home cooked meal and having to rush through it. While it may seem like this is not going to be hard to do, arranging meals around vegetables will be a foreign concept for many people and it will take them several minutes to do and to get right the first time. Give yourself plenty of time to do this and you will be able to create hearty and delicious meals that will leave you feeling satisfied.

3. Avoid Any Type of Convenience Food

If you are skeptical about how delicious or savory vegan dishes can be, I highly recommend that you stay away from as many vegan convenience food products as possible. Trust me, I have yet to taste one that has been good and that I liked really well. If you think that you will be able to live on frozen pizza, frozen vegan burritos and veggie burger patties every single day, you are going to be in one heck of a surprise.

4. Do Not Be Embarrassed About Living This Kind of Lifestyle

There may come a time where you will feel that you have to rationalize your decision or explain your decision to other people. You may even find yourself coming up with reasons behind your Vegan lifestyle such as, "I'm doing it as a research project or I didn't want to hurt animals." Regardless of what reason you are using, you will begin to notice the same thing happening over and over again: explaining yourself never feels good.

Never feel that you have to explain your decision to anybody. However, if you do want something to tell people I find it easy to come out and say, "I have always agreed with Vegan philosophy and this just felt right." Most people have nothing to say to that statement. In fact most people will become more intrigued and you will find yourself having an interesting discussion with people that you may or may not know.

5. If You Mess Up, Don't Beat Yourself Up Over It

Let's face it, none of us are perfect. There may be a couple of times when you may accidentally consume some butter with animal fat or accidentally had something with fish sauce in it. Unfortunately this happens more than you may like and if it happens to happen to you, do not beat yourself up about it.

If you are stuck somewhere whether it is your home or out on the road and you have no choice, but to consume something with a hint of animal in it then do it and do not beat yourself up over it in the long run. You will have to make mistakes every now and then while on this diet and your time could be better spent learning from these mistakes then letting them hold you back.

6. Don't Be Afraid of The Produce Isle

Going Vegan means that you will get to become close and personal with the produce isle then you may have been before. Once you start this diet is a good idea to head down this isle to learn and explore exactly what your new diet will begin to consist of. Look at how much diversity you have with plants and try to come up with some creative meal ideas while surrounded by the main ingredients that you will be using.

7. Stay As Strong As You Possibly Can

Going Vegan is not the easiest thing that you will ever do. In fact, it will be one of the hardest things that you will do. The first few days will be especially tough on you, but I promise it does become easier as days pass. You will soon get into the swing of things and living this lifestyle will become easier and easier. It will come to a point that when you think of what you want to make for every meal, meat will never cross your mind.

8. There Are Plenty of Places To Eat Out At That Offer Healthy Vegan Options

Just because you are Vegan does not mean that you cannot indulge yourself on delicious food every once in a while. There are many restaurants that you can go to and till enjoy yourself such as Moe's Mexican restaurant, Johnny Rockets, Chipotle and P.F. Changs. If your friends ever want to go out and do something with you that involves eating, do not be afraid to suggest one of these popular restaurants.

9. Get On a Vitamin B12 Supplement

As discussed in the first chapter of this eBook, most Vegans tend to suffer from the same common ailment, which is Vitamin B12 deficiency. In order to reduce the risk of getting this ailment and to ensure that you feel as healthy as possible begin taking a Vitamin B12 supplement as soon as you begin this lifestyle. Trust me, you will not regret it in the long run.

10. When In Doubt, Stick With Simplicity

Just because you are a Vegan and you are using vegetables to make up the majority of your meals, it does not mean that you have to make the entire process complicated. The best recipes to make are the simple ones and not only will you enjoy these recipes, but so will your guests.

If you are just starting out on a Vegan Diet, these helpful tips will help you to become a successful Vegan in the long run. Whether you ensure to explore your options when eating out, staying as strong as possible with your new lifestyle, having an open mind about being a Vegan, making sure that you stay clear of Vegan convenience foods and making sure to give yourself plenty of time to prepare your meals, make sure that you try to follow these tips every once in a while. You will become a better Vegan for it in the long run.

Chapter 3: Five Ways To Make Your Vegan Meals Taste Amazing

When it comes to eating a Vegan diet most of the time people are hesitant about it. Why is this? The main reason people are resistant to the idea of eating a healthy Vegan diet is because many people are under the misconception that the food will not taste as good as a burger and fries will. This is one of the most popular misconceptions regarding a Vegan diet today and in my opinion it is one that stops many people from becoming great Vegans and from living a healthier lifestyle in the long run.

When you first begin preparing Vegan food, many people do not know how to make their dishes tastes good. There are so many different flavors to work with that bringing them out so that you can savor them can be extremely difficult. There are many different seasoning that you can use to bring out the flavor of your dish and to help impress not only yourself, but your friends and family as well.

Here are 5 different tips that you can use to help make your vegan meals taste more amazing and to get you excited to prepare your meals on a daily basis.

1. Make Sure That You Use Only High-Quality and Fresh Ingredients

One of the best ways to ensure that your food tastes just as delicious as possible is to ensure that you are using the highest quality ingredients that you can afford and that you are as fresh as possible.

If you are the type of person who usually only spends enough money to get the cheapest ingredients possible, you will begin to notice that you meals are lacking in flavor, making it more possible that you will stop your Vegan diet before you want to.

I highly recommend using fresh organic ingredients, as they always tend to pack more punch then ordinary produce. Keep in mind, the ingredients that are simple and that are not stuffed with things like salt and sugar, have more flavor and will help your meals to taste delicious in the long run.

2. Don't Be Afraid To Spice Things Up

Using different herbs and spices should start becoming a regular part of your meal preparing process and it is something that you should get in the habit of adding into your meals on a daily basis. Not only do herbs and spices help to add incredible flavor to your meals, but many of them are packed with important nutrients that your body needs on a daily basis.

Some of the most popular and great tasting spices that you can use are turmeric, cinnamon, cumin and ginger. These four spices can help liven up a dull vegan dish and can even help benefit your body in the long run such as by giving your digestive system a boost that it desperately needs.

Using fresh herbs in your dishes can also help give your body important antioxidants and nutrients that it needs. Herbs like Parsley, cilantro, Basil and Mint can be used for much more then great tasting garnishes and you can use them for a variety of reasons in your main dishes.

3. When Using Beans and Grains, Give Them A Boost Once In A While

If you have ever eaten plain chickpeas or brown rice, you know better than anybody how unappealing they can be. They are completely bland and don't really have much of a taste to them. If you are making a dish that must incorporate these two ingredients, I highly recommend that you do not serve them on their own.

I highly recommend pairing your beans and grains with ingredients that are rich in flavor. Try mixing them with some of your favorite pieces of fruit. There are even some vegetables that you can use that can help liven up the flavors of these otherwise bland foods.

I also recommend adding a healthy helping of flavorful sauce or dressing to some of these ingredients.

4. Don't Be Afraid To Use Fat In Your Meals

While choosing the right kind of fat to use in your dish is important to keep your meals and yourself as healthy as possible, the more you do it, the easier the process becomes down the line. Adding healthy forms of fat not only have healthy benefits for you, but it can go a long way into making your meals much more delicious. Fat carries the richness of the entire dish and can make or break how the dish will taste to you and your family.

There are many types of healthy fat that you can use to enhance the flavor of your dish such as fats coming from whole foods like seeds, avocados, olives and nuts. If you find that you are preparing a meal for other people who are following the Vegan lifestyle as well, it will help to add a healthy form of fat to enhance the taste of dish.

5. Don't Be Afraid To Use Salt Here and There

Salt helps out to bring out the flavor of important vegan ingredients such as vegetables and even helps to soften them a bit whenever you are cooking them up or sautéing them. When you are preparing your meals do not be afraid to add as much salt as you want to help bring out the flavor of your veggies.

If you are afraid of taking in too much sodium there are healthy alternatives that you can use to help enhance the flavor of your dishes. Don't be afraid to use vegetable salt every once in a while as it contains lots of important nutrients and less sodium than regular table salt.

I know that starting a Vegan diet can be very scary and can even feel intimidating when you do not believe that you will be able to eat delicious meals again. However, there are certain things that you can do to enhance the flavors of your dishes such as using salt, healthy forms of fat or using fruits to bring out the flavors of your dishes. Follow these helpful tips to make the most delicious Vegan recipes you will ever make in your life.

Vegan Breakfast Recipes

Lemon Scones Vegan Style

This delicious recipe is one that every Vegan should try. With this recipe you can feel free to be as creative as you want and you can experiment as much as you like as well.

Total Prep Time: 25 Minutes

Serves: 12

Ingredients:
- ¾ Cup of Sugar, White
- 4 tsp. of Baking Powder
- ½ tsp. Salt
- ¾ Cup of Margarine, Slightly Melted
- 2 Cups of Flour, All Purpose
- ½ Cup of Water
- 2 Tbsp. of Poppy Seeds
- 1 Lemon, Used For Juice and Zest
- ½ Cup of Soy Milk

Directions:
1. Preheat your oven to 400 degrees. While it heats up grease a small baking sheet and set aside.

2. In a large mixing bowl combine your sugar, flour, salt and baking powder until thoroughly combined. Add in your margarine and cut it into your mixture until it has the consistency of sand. Then stir in your lemon juice, poppy seeds and lemon zest.
3. Next add in your soymilk and water together and stir with your dry ingredients until your mixture slowly becomes a batter that is thick. It should resemble biscuit dough.
4. Then spoon small amounts of your dough onto your greased baking sheet and ensure that your scones are about 3 inches apart from each other.
5. Place Into Your Oven and bake for the next 10 to 15 minutes until they are golden brown in color. Remove from oven and place on cooling rack to cool before serving.

Blueberry and Cornmeal Pancakes

When you make these pancakes, you will never have to worry about breaking your vegan diet at all. These pancakes tastes extremely great with some warmed blueberry jam or your favorite brand of syrup.

Total Prep Time: 25 Minutes

Serves: 4

Ingredients:
- 1 Cup of Soymilk
- ¼ tsp. of Salt For Taste
- 1 Cup of Flour, Whole Wheat
- ½ Cup of Water
- 1 tsp. of Baking Powder
- ½ tsp. of Baking Soda
- 1 Cup of Blueberries, Fresh
- 2 Tbsp. of Vegetable Oil
- **½ Cup of Cornmeal, Ground**

Directions:
1. Preheat your oven to 200 degrees. While it heats up take out a small mixing bowl and combine your water and soy milk into it.
2. In a separate mixing bowl combine your dry ingredients together: baking powder, flour, baking soda, flour and

salt until all ingredients are thoroughly mixed. Then stir in your soymilk and water mixture to your dry ingredients. As you continue to stir fold in your fresh blueberries gently and stir until well mixed. Allow your batter to sit for at least 5 minutes.

3. Grab a skillet and lightly grease it with a generous amount of cooking spray. Heat it over medium heat and then pour about ¼ cup of batter into your skillet. Cook gently until bubbles begin to form on the top of your pancake and flip it. Allow to cook on the other side for about 3 to 5 minutes. Remove from skillet and place on a baking sheet. Place the baking sheet into your oven and allow your pancakes to remain warm while you cook the rest of your batter.

Vegan Style Crepes

Crepes are absolutely delicious and many people who are on a vegan diet often wonder if they can even enjoy this excellent breakfast dish. Well, now you no longer need to worry as this crepe recipe has a classic vegan style twist on it. Not only will this recipe taste great, but it will leave you wanting more.

Total Prep Time: 2 ½ Hours

Serves: 4

Ingredients:
- ½ Cup of Water
- 1 Tbsp. of Sugar, Turbinado
- ½ Cup of Soymilk
- ¼ tsp. of Salt, For Taste
- 2 Tbsp. of Syrup
- 1 Cup of Flour, Unbleached and All Purpose
- **¼ Cup of Soy Margarine, Melted**

Directions:
1. In a large mixing bowl combine your soymilk, water, syrup, salt, margarine and water together until thoroughly mixed. Cover your mixture with some plastic wrap and allow to chill in your refrigerate for at least 2 hours.

2. Take out a medium sized skillet and lightly grease it with some soy margarine over medium to high heat. Pour about 3 Tbsp. of your chilled batter into your skillet and swirl around to ensure your batter covers the entire bottom of the skillet. Cook your crepe until golden in color an flip to cook on the opposite side..

Breakfast Style Raisin and Rice Pudding

With this recipe you can finally find a way to put your leftover rice to good use. Feel free to serve this dish while hot or cold. Either way it will taste great.

Total Prep Time: 20 Minutes

Serves: 4

Ingredients:
- 1 Cup of Soymilk
- 1 Cup of Water
- ½ Cup of Raisins
- ¼ Cup of Syrup Of Your Choice
- 1 tsp. of Cinnamon, Ground

- ½ Cup of Almonds, Toasted and Chopped Finely
- 3 Cups of Brown Rice, Fully Cooked
- **½ tsp. of Cardamom, Ground**

Directions:

1. In a small mixing bowl combine your raisins, soymilk, cardamom, cooked rice, chopped almonds, syrup and cinnamon. Place into a pot over medium to high heat and allow to come to a boil.
2. Once it comes to a boil reduce the heat to low and allow your pudding to simmer for the next 5 to 8 minutes. Remove from heat and serve into small bowls.

Breakfast Strawberry and Oatmeal

Smoothie

This rich vegan smoothie is extremely filling and will surely satisfy any food cravings that you may have. It is pink in color and contains a creamy texture that will leave you wanting more.

Total Prep Time: 5 Minutes

Serves: 2

Ingredients:
- 1 Cup of Milk, Soy
- 14 Strawberries, Fresh or Frozen
- ½ tsp. of Vanilla Extract
- ½ Cup of Oats, Rolled
- 1 ½ tsp. of Sugar, White
- **1 Banana, Peeled and Cut Into Small Chunks**

Directions:
1. In a blender, combine all of your ingredients together and blend on the lowest setting until if reaches the desired consistency. Pour into small glasses and serve immediately.

Vegan Style Apple and Carrot Breakfast Muffins

This is the perfect recipe to make if you want to impress your family or friends at the office. This recipe makes plenty of muffins that are incredibly delicious and that are healthy for you.

Total Prep Time: 40 Minutes

Serves: 12

Ingredients:
- 1 Cup of Brown Sugar
- 4 tsp. of Cinnamon, Ground
- ½ Cup of Sugar, White
- 1 tsp. of Baking Powder
- 2 ½ Cups of Flour, All-Purpose
- 4 tsp. of Baking Soda
- 6 tsp. of Egg Replacer, Dry
- 2 tsp. of Salt
- ¼ Cup of Vegetable Oil
- 2 Cups of Carrots, Finely Grated
- 2 Apples, Large In Size, Peeled, Cored and Shredded Finely
- **1 ¼ Cups of Applesauce**

Directions:
1. Preheat your oven to 375 degrees. As it heats up grease a muffin tin lightly or line it some muffin liners

2. In a large sized mixing bowl combine your baking soda, white sugar, cinnamon, brown sugar, flour, salt and baking powder together and stir until all of the ingredients are thoroughly combined.
3. In a small sized mixing bowl whisk together your applesauce, oil and dry egg substitute until all of the ingredients are mixed completely. Then stir this into your dry ingredients until thoroughly mixed.
4. Spoon some batter generously into your greased muffin pan at least ¾ of the way full for each muffin tin.
5. Place into your oven and bake for the next 20 minutes. Remove from oven and allow your muffins to cool for about 5 minutes before trying to remove your muffins from the pan.

Healthy Banana and Kale Smoothie

This smoothie is rich in important nutrients that your body craves on a daily basis. While it does contain kale, the flavor of the banana hides it completely, leaving you with a smoothie that you will simple love.

Total Prep Time: 5 Minutes

Serves: 1

Ingredients:

- 1 Banana, Peeled and Cut Into Small Chunks
- 2 Cups of Kale, Chopped
- 1 Tbsp. of Flaxseeds
- 1 tsp. of Syrup, Maple
- **½ Cup of Soymilk, Unsweetened and Light**

Directions:

1. Place all over your ingredients into a blender and blend until the smoothie reaches the consistency that you like. Pour into a drinking glass and serve immediately.

Classic Oat Bran Cereal

If you need a dish that you can make fast and that is relatively easy to make, this is the perfect recipe for you. This hot breakfast recipe is sweetened with sugar substitute and some dried plums, making it a nutritious and delicious recipe.

Total Prep Time: 10 Minutes

Serves: 1

Ingredients:
- 1 Cup of Water, Warm
- 5 Dried Prunes, Chopped Into Small Pieces
- ¼ Cup of Oat Bran
- ¼ tsp. of Cinnamon, Ground
- **1 tsp. of Sugar Substitute, Splenda**

Directions:
1. In a small to medium sized saucepan, combine your prunes, splenda, water and cinnamon together. Heat over low to medium heat until it reaches a boil.
2. Then stir in your oat bran and allow to boil for the next 2 minutes. Remove from heat and serve immediately.

Vegan Lunch Recipes

Spicy Lentil Wraps

A great recipe to help wake you up right in the middle of the day. This dish is really easy to make and will leave you feeling full for the rest of the day.
Total Prep Time: 60 Minutes
Serves: 6
Ingredients For Wraps:
- 2 Cups of Water, Warm
- ¾ Cups of Bulgur, Fine Grain
- ½ Cup of Lentils, Red and Rinsed
- 2 tsp. of Cumin, Ground
- 2 Tbsp. of Olive Oil
- ½ tsp. of Salt
- 1 Scallion, Chopped Finely
- 1 tsp. of Red Pepper Flakes
- 2 Cubs of Cabbage, Shredded

- 2 Tbsp. of Parsley, Fresh and Finely Chopped
- ¾ Cup of Red Pepper Paste
- **6 Sheet of Lavish, Whole Wheat or White**

Ingredients For Tahini Sauce:
- ¼ Cup of Tahini
- 2 tsp. of Lemon Juice, Fresh
- ¼ tsp. of Garlic, Crushed
- 1/8 tsp. of Salt
- 2/3 Cup of Warm Water
- 1/8 tsp. of Red Pepper Flakes
- **2 tsp. of Parsley, Fresh and Finely Chopped**

1. Directions For Wraps:

In a small saucepan over medium heat, combine both your lentils and your water together. Allow the water to boil then reduce the water to a small simmer. Allow your lentils to simmer for about 20 minutes or until they become soft.

Remove from heat and stir in your bulgur and all to sit with your water and lentils for about 30 minutes or until it becomes soft.

While the bulgur sits, heat some oil in a medium sized saucepan. Sauté your onions, red pepper flakes and cumin together until the onions are translucent. Once soft add this mixture to your bulgur mixture and stir until all of the ingredients are thoroughly combined.

To assemble lay out one sheet of lavish and put together like a burrito. Wait to wrap it up until the tahini sauce.

Directions For Tahini Sauce:

1. In a small sized mixing combine all of your ingredients together and stir with a form until all of the ingredients are combined thoroughly.
2. Then gradually add some warm water to it until the sauce reaches the consistency that you are looking for and serve about 1 Tbsp. with your lentil wraps.

Delicious Quinoa Salad With Fresh Avocado and Dill

What lunch is completely without a salad. If you haven't gotten the chance to try Quinoa yet, this recipe will help you fall in love with it. Feel free to be creative as you want with this recipe and add in whatever additional vegan friendly ingredients that you want.

Total Prep Time: 30 Minutes
Serves: 4 to 6
Ingredients:
- 1 Cup of Quinoa, Golden
- 1 Shallot, Large In Size and Chopped Finely
- 1 ¾ Cups of Vegetable Broth
- 8 Radishes, Small In Size and Chopped Finely
- 2/3 Cups of Dill, Stems Gone
- 3 Tbsp. of Olive Oil, Extra Virgin
- ½ Tbsp. of Vinegar, Balsamic
- ½ Cup of Almonds, Sliced Finely
- ½ Cup of Dates, Chopped Roughly

- ½ Lemon, Fresh and Used From Juice and Zest
- 1/3 of a Cucumber, Sliced Thinly
- Dash of Salt and Pepper For Taste
- 1 Avocado, Ripe and Cut Into Small Chunks

Directions:

1. Rinse your quinoa while using a fine mesh strainer for at least 2 to 3 minutes, making sure to rub the quinoa vigorously while you are doing it.
2. In a medium sized saucepan heat up your extra virgin olive oil and cook your quinoa in the oil for about 1 to 2 minutes. Then pour in your vegetable broth and allow to come to a boil. Once it does turn the heat down to the lowest setting and allow to cook for about 15 minutes. After 15 minutes remove from heat and allow to sit for 5 minutes.
3. Drain your quinoa and place into a bowl to allow to cool completely.
4. Place your remaining ingredients into a small sized mixing bowl and toss until all of the ingredients are thoroughly

combined. Toss in your quinoa and stir until well mixed.
5. Serve into a salad bowl and enjoy immediately.

Vegan Style Mac and Cheese

Nobody said that even as a vegan, you cannot enjoy mac and cheese every once in a while. Even though cheese is definitely on the list of things that you naturally can't have, this recipe will leave you a dish that you will certainly crave on a daily basis.

Total Prep Time: 1 Hour and 15 Minutes
Serves: 4
Ingredients:
- 3 Tbsp. of Yeast, Nutritional Kind
- 1 Pack of Macaroni, Elbow Kind and Uncooked
- 1 Onion, Medium In Size, Finely Chopped
- 1 Tbsp. of Vegetable Oil
- 1/3 Cup of Lemon Juice, Fresh

- 1 1/3 Cups of Warm Water
- 1 Cup of Cashews, Finely Chopped
- 1/3 Cup of Canola Oil
- Dash of Salt and Pepper For Taste
- 1 tsp. of Garlic Powder
- 1 tsp. of Onion Powder
- 4 Ounces of Red Peppers, Roasted and Drained

Directions:

1. Preheat your oven to 350 degrees.
2. While your oven heats up, cook up your elbow macaroni until it is al dente. Once your drain it transfer it to a medium sized baking dish.
3. In a medium sized saucepan, sauté your onions over low to medium heat or until they are softened and lightly brown in color. Remove from heat and mix in with your macaroni in the baking dish.
4. Using a food processor put your lemon juice, cashews, salt and some water and mix up until it reaches a fine consistency. Then toss in the remainder of your ingredients and blend until smooth. Pour this in with your

macaroni and onions and stir until all of the ingredients are mixed well.
5. Place into your oven and bake for 45 minutes until your macaroni is lightly brown. Remove from your oven and allow to cool for at least 10 to 15 minutes before you serve it.

Hearty Zucchini and Red Pepper Stew

This dish will satisfy you unlike any other vegan dish that you come across. It is hearty and savory, making this a dish that you will want to make all of the time.

Total Prep Time: 1 Hour and 20 Minutes
Serves: 4 Servings
Ingredients:
- ¼ Cup of Olive Oil
- ½ Cup of Rice, Basmati
- 1 Eggplant, Sliced Into 1 Inch Cubes
- 5 Cloves of Garlic, Chopped Finely
- 3 Tomatoes, Fresh and Diced Into Small Pieces
- 1 Cup of Onions, Chopped Finely
- 1 Red Bell pepper, Chopped Into Small Pieces

- 1 ½ Cups of Water, Warm
- ¼ tsp. of Red Pepper Flakes
- ¼ Cup of Basil, Fresh
- ½ tsp. of Salt and Pepper For Taste
- ¼ Cup of Parsley, Fresh and Chopped Finely
- 1 Sprig of Rosemary, Fresh and Chopped
- **1 Cup of Wine, Marsala**

Directions:

1. Place your eggplant into a medium sized colander and sprinkle with your dash of salt and pepper. Slice up your eggplant and sauté in a pan with some oil until it is slightly brown in color. Then stir in your onion and sauté until the onions are translucent. Next add in your garlic and sauté with your eggplant and onion for about 2 to 3 minutes.

2. Then stir in your rice, tomatoes, water, red pepper flakes, some additional salt, pepper, zucchini and red bell pepper. Make sure your cook your mixture over medium heat until it reaches a nice rolling boil and then reduce the heat.

Allow to simmer for about 45 minutes or until all of your vegetables are tender.
3. Remove from heat and stir in your rosemary, basil and parsley until thoroughly combined. Serve while still piping hot.

Vegan Style Black Bean Quesadillas

These quesadillas pack quite a punch and will leave you feel exceptionally full. You can gorge all your want without feeling guilty about consuming cheese.

Total Prep Time: 55 Minutes

Serves: 4

Ingredients:
- 1 Clove of Garlic, Minced
- 1 Can of Northern Beans, Drained and Rinsed Prior to Use
- ¼ tsp. of Chili Powder
- ¾ Cup of Tomatoes, Diced
- 1 tsp. of Cumin, Ground
- 1/3 Cup of Yeast, Nutritional
- ¼ Cup of Tomatoes, Diced Finely
- 1 Pinch of Cayenne Pepper

- 1 Tbsp. of Olive Oil
- Some Cooking Spray
- 8 Tortillas, Whole Grain
- ½ Cup of Vegan Black Beans, Drained and Rinsed
- Dash of Salt and Pepper For Tastes

Directions:

1. Using a food processor blend up your Northern beans, garlic and ¾ cup of diced tomatoes until it reaches a smooth consistency. Then add in your cumin, salt, pepper, chili powder, red pepper flakes and nutritional yeast until thoroughly mixed and smooth.
2. Transfer your mixture to a bowl and then stir in your black beans and ¼ cup of diced Tomatoes. Stir until thoroughly mixed.
3. Heat some olive oil over medium heat in a medium sized saucepan. Place one tortilla into your saucepan and fill the middle with a generous amount of bean filling. Place a second tortilla on top of your filling and allow to cook for about 10 minutes.

4. Spray the top of your quesadilla with some cooking spray and flip to allow to cook on the other side for about 6 to 7 minutes. Slide onto a plate and serve immediately.

Scrambled Up Tofu

If you are looking to enjoy a high protein meal to help bring some enjoyment in your day, you are going to love this recipe. Feel free to add spinach, cashews or mushrooms to this dish as a topping.

Total Prep Time: 25 Minutes

Serves: 4

Ingredients:

- 1 Onion, Medium In Size and Chopped Finely
- 1 Tbsp. of Olive Oil
- 3 Cloves of Garlic, Minced
- ½ Can of Black Olives, Drained and Cut Into halves
- 1 Pack of Tofu, Drained and Cut Into Cubes
- 1 Tbsp. of Soy Sauce
- 3 Tbsp. of Yeast, Nutritional

Directions:
1. Using a cast iron skillet, heat up some oil over low to medium heat, cook your onion until they are softened. This should take about 5 to 10 minutes. Then add in your tofu, olives and garlic. Cover your skillet and allow to cook for an additional 8 minutes, stirring every once in a while.
2. Then add in your yeast and soy sauces. Stir until your yeast fully dissolves which should take about 1 to 2 minutes.

Asian Style Lettuce Wraps

This dish is packed with delicious veggies, crunchy vegetables and fresh ginger. This dish is not only very colorful, but it tastes great as well.

Total Prep Time: 22 Minutes
Serves: 8 Wraps
Ingredients:
- 2 tsp. of Canola Oil

- 1 Clove of Garlic, Minced
- 2 Tbsp. of Hoisin Sauce
- 1 Pinch of Red Chili Peppers, Dried
- 2 tsp. of Gingerroot, Grated Finely
- ½ tsp. of Sesame Oil
- A few Leaves of Lettuce
- 1/3 Cup of Coriander, Fresh and Chopped Finely
- 1/3 Cup of Green Onion, Chopped Finely
- ½ Cup of Cucumber, Diced Into Thin Pieces
- ½ Cup of Carrot, Shredded
- ½ Cup of Red Pepper, Sweet and Diced Into Small Pieces

Directions:

1. In a large sized non-stick skillet, heat up some oil over low to medium heat. Add in your garlic and gingerroot and allow to cook for the next 2 minutes or until they become soft and light brown in color.
2. Next stir in your sesame oil and hoisin sauce. Add in your chili peppers and stir until well mixed. Reduce your heat to

the lowest setting and cook for the next 5 minutes.
3. Remove from heat and lay out your lettuce wraps on a flat surface. Take about 3 Tbsp. of your vegetable filling onto each leaf of lettuce and wrap like a burrito. Enjoy.

Classic Chickpea Curry

While this is an easy recipe to make, it allows you to be as creative as you want with it. Do not hesitate to spice up the ingredients a bit especially if you usually make this dish as frequently as possible.

Total Prep Time: 40 Minutes
Serves: 8
Ingredients:
- 2 Onions, Minced
- 2 Tbsp. of Vegetable Oil
- 1 tsp. of Cumin, Ground
- 6 Cloves, Whole
- 2 Cloves of Garlic, Minced
- 1 tsp. of Coriander, Ground
- Dash of Salt and Pepper For Taste
- 1 Cup of Cilantro, Fresh

- 1 tsp. of Cayenne Pepper
- 1 tsp. of Turmeric, Ground
- 2, 15 Ounce Cans of Garbanzo Beans
- 2 Sticks of Cinnamon, Crushed
- 2 tsp. of Ginger Root, Fresh and Chopped Finely

Directions:

1. Using a large frying pan, heat up some oil in it and fry your onions until they are tender.
2. Stir in the remainder of your ingredients and allow to cook for about 30 to 35 minutes. Remove from heat and stir in your cilantro just before serving. Enjoy.

Vegan Dinner Recipes

Vegan Style Fajitas

This recipe is the most wonderful version of meatless fajitas that you can make. It make enough that you can prepare it ahead of time or save a little extra for your friends and family.

Total Prep Time: 1 Hour and 10 Minutes
Serves: 6
Ingredients:
- ¼ Cup of Vinegar, Red Wine
- 1 tsp. of Sugar, White
- ¼ Cup of Olive Oil
- 1 tsp. of Chili Powder
- 1 tsp. of Oregano, Dried
- Dash of Salt, Garlic Salt and Pepper For Taste
- 2 Zucchini, Small In Size and Slice Julienne Style
- 1 Onion, Large In Size, Sliced Into Small Pieces
- 1 Yellow Squash, Small In Size and Sliced Julienne Style
- 2 Tbsp. of Olive Oil
- 1, 15 Ounce Can of Black Beans, Drained and Rinsed
- 1, 8 Ounce Can of Corn, Whole Kernel and Drained
- 1 Red Bell Pepper, Cut Into Thin Strips
- 1 Green Bell Pepper, Cut Into Thin Strips

Directions:
1. In a medium sized mixing bowl combine your oregano, garlic salt, salt, sugar, pepper, olive oil, vinegar and chili powder until well mixed. Then add in your onion, squash and peppers to the marinade and stir until thoroughly mixed. Place in your fridge for at least 30 minutes.
2. Heat up a large sized skillet over low to medium heat. Add in your drained vegetables and sauté all of them until they are tender. This should take about 10 to 15 minutes. Then stir in your beans and corn and cook over high heat for at least 5 minutes. Serve while still piping hot.

Vegan Style Spicy Potato Curry

If you have ever been bored of curry, this recipe will change your mind. This recipe helps to bring a little spice and flavor into a traditional curry dish that you will fall in love with.

Total Prep Time: 60 Minutes

Serves: 6

Ingredients:
- 4 tsp. of Curry Powder
- 4 Potatoes, Washed, Peeled and Cut Into Small Cubes
- 2 Tbsp. of Vegetable Oil
- 3 Cloves of Garlic, Minced
- 1 ½ tsp. of Cayenne Pepper
- 1 Onion, Yellow In Color and Diced Into Small Chunks
- 2 tsp. of Cumin, Ground
- 2 tsp. of Salt
- 4 tsp. of Garam Masala
- 1 Ginger Root, Peeled and Minced
- 1, 14 Ounce Can of Tomatoes, Diced Into Small Chunks
- 1, 14 Ounce Can of Coconut Milk
- 1, 15 Ounce Can of Peas, Drained
- 1, 15 Ounce Can of Chickpeas, Drained and Rinsed

Directions:
1. Place your potatoes into a large sized pot over high heat. Place some salt into it with your potatoes and allow your potatoes to boil for about 15 minutes or until they become tender. Drain your

potatoes and let them dry out by themselves for about a minute or two.
2. Then using a large non-stick skillet, sauté your onions and garlic in some vegetable oil over medium heat. Sauté until the onions become translucent in color, which should take about 5 minutes. Then season your sautéed veggies with some curry powder, salt, ginger, garam masala, cumin and cayenne pepper.
3. Next add in your tomatoes, peas, potatoes, garbanzo beans and coconut milk and stir until thoroughly blended. Allow your mixture to simmer for 5 to 10 minutes and then serve while still piping hot.

Delicious Avocado Tacos

These tacos are simple and easy to make and taste amazing as well. You will want to make this dish all of the time.

Total Prep Time: 25 Minutes

Serves: 6

Ingredients:

- ¼ Cup of Onions, Diced Into Small Pieces
- 3 Avocados, Peeled, Pitted and Mashed Into A Smooth Consistency
- ¼ tsp. of Garlic Salt
- Dash of Jalapeno Pepper Sauce, For Taste
- 12 Corn Tortillas
- Some Fresh Leaves of Cilantro, Chopped Finely

Directions:

1. Preheat your oven to 325 degrees.
2. While your oven heats up, take out a medium sized mixing bowl. In the bowl mix up your garlic salt, avocado and onions until it reaches a smooth consistency.

3. Then arrange your tortillas on a greased baking sheet and place into your oven for 2 to 5 minutes so that they are heated through. Then spread your avocado mixture onto your tortillas and garnish with some fresh cilantro and jalapeno pepper sauce. Serve immediately.

Traditional Vegan Quinoa Chard Pilaf

This incredibly simple vegan dish combines a variety of delicious ingredients that you will surely love. It also is very colorful, which will surely even please the pickiest of eaters.

Total Prep Time: 40 Minutes

Serves: 8

Ingredients:
- 1 Onion, Medium In Size and Diced Into Small Pieces
- 1 Tbsp. of Olive Oil
- 3 Cloves of Garlic, Minced
- 2 Cups of Quinoa, Uncooked and Rinsed
- 1 Quart of Vegetable Broth

- 1 Cup of Lentils, Canned and Rinsed
- 1 Bunch of Swiss Chard, Stems Cut
- 8 Ounces of Mushrooms, Chopped Finely

Directions:

1. In a medium sized pan, heat up some oil over low to medium heat. Pour your chopped onion and garlic into the pan and sauté for about 5 minutes or until the onion becomes tender. Mix in your quinoa, mushrooms and lentils. Stir thoroughly until completely combined.
2. Next pour in your vegetable broth and cover. Allow to simmer for about 20 minutes.
3. Remove your pot from heat and gently mix in your Swiss chard. Cover again and let your mixture sit for 5 minutes or until it is fully wilted.

Vegan Style Shepherd's Pie

Even though following a Vegan diet can be tough, it does not mean that you can't still enjoy recipes you love. With this recipe you will be able to enjoy a meatless shepherd's pie that tastes great

Total Prep Time: 1 Hour and 15 Minutes
Serves: 8
Ingredients:
- Dash of Salt and Pepper For Taste
- 2 Cups of Vegetable Broth, Divide Into 2, 1 Cup Servings
- ½ Cup of Lentils, Dry
- 1 Carrot, Large In Size and Diced Into Fine Pieces
- ½ of an Onion, Chopped Finely
- ¼ Cup of Barley, Pearl
- 1 tsp. of Yeast Extract
- ½ tsp. of Water
- 3 Potatoes, Chopped Into Small Pieces
- ½ Cup of Walnuts, Chopped Coarsely
- 1 tsp. of Flour, All Purpose

Directions:
1. Preheat your oven to 350 degrees.
2. Using a large sized saucepan over low to medium heat add in your broth, lentils, barley and yeast extract and stir until mixed. Allow to simmer for about 30 minutes.

3. In a separate medium sized saucepan, bring together your vegetable broth, walnuts, onions and carrots and allow to cook until the vegetables are still tender. This should take about 15 minutes.
4. In another separate pot, bring some water and salt together and bring to a boil. Place your potatoes into this pot and allow them to cook over medium to high heat for 15 minutes or until they become tender. Once tender drain the potatoes and mashed them until they reach the consistency you want.
5. Add in your flour and water to your carrot mixture and stir until thoroughly combined. Combine your carrot mixture with your lentil mixture next and season with as much salt and pepper as you like. Pour this mixture into a baking dish and place into your oven for about 30 minutes or until the top is nice and brown. Remove from oven and serve while still piping hot.

Mediterranean Zucchini

If you are a fan of Mediterranean cuisine then you are going to love this recipe. Feel free to serve this dish over a side of rice or nutritious egg noodles to make the perfect dinner meal.

Total Prep Time: 60 Minutes
Serves: 6
Ingredients:
- 3 Cloves of Garlic, Crushed and Minced
- 2 Cups of Water
- 3 Tbsp. of Olive Oil
- 1 Red Bell Pepper, Finely Chopped
- 1 Onion, Large In Size and Chopped Finely
- 1 Cup of White Rice, Long Grain
- Dash of Salt and Pepper For Taste
- 1, 14 Ounce Can of Tomatoes, Peeled and Chopped Finely
- 3 Cups of Zucchini, Chopped Into Small Pieces
- ½ tsp. of Oregano, Dried
- 1, 15 Ounce Can of Cannellini Beans, Drained and Rinsed

Directions:

1. In a medium sized saucepan, bring some water oven medium heat and stir in your rice. Allow to simmer for about 20 minutes until it is fully cooked.
2. In another saucepan, heat up some oil over low to medium heat. Stir in your garlic, onion and red bell pepper. Stir consistently until the mixture becomes fully tender. Mix in your tomatoes and zucchini next. Season with some salt, pepper and oregano and cover your skillet. Reduce your heat and allow to simmer for the next 20 minutes, making sure to stir as frequently as possible.
3. Then stir in your bean to your mixture and let cook for an additional 10 minutes. Once done serve over your cooked rice and enjoy.

Delicious Tomato Pasta

This is an extremely simple recipe to make and you will want to make it as frequently as possible. Feel free to use whatever kind of pasta that you like.

Total Prep Time: 22 Minutes

Serves: 2

Ingredients:

- 1 Tomato, Medium In Size and Coarsely Chopped
- 1 Clove of Garlic, Coarsely Chopped
- Dash of Salt and Pepper For Taste
- 1 tsp. of Basil, Dried
- 1 Tbsp. of Olive Oil
- 1 Package of Pasta of Your Choice, Dried

Directions:

1. Cook your pasta thoroughly in a large pot of boiling water. Cook until pasta is al dente, drain and set aside to use later.
2. In a small mixing bowl combine your tomatoes, basil, olive oil and salt. Toss until all of the ingredients are

thoroughly mixed. Pour over your cooked pasta and serve. Enjoy.

Teriyaki Style Tofu With Pineapple

You would be surprised by how well tofu and teriyaki work well together. This dish has a bit of spice and tang that you will fall in love with.

Total Prep Time: 1 Hour and 25 Minutes
Serves: 4
Ingredients:

- 2 Cups of Teriyaki Sauce, Your Favorite Kind
- 1 Pack of Tofu, Firm
- 1 Cup of Pineapple, Fresh and Chopped Into Small Chunks

Directions:

1. Slice up your tofu until you have a bunch of bite sized pieces and place them into a baking dish. Add in your pineapple and teriyaki sauce and mix until the tofu is evenly coated. Place into your fridge for at least 1 hour.
2. Preheat your oven to 350 degrees and upon being chilled for an hour place

your dish into your oven. Allow to bake for 20 minutes or until the dish is piping hot and bubbly. Remove and serve immediately.

Vegan Desserts

Vegan Style Cupcakes

I know that giving up anything ingredient made from animals can be quite difficult at times, it is not at all impossible to enjoy great tasting desserts. This recipe will help you make the most delicious cupcakes you will ever make and they taste just like the real thing.

Total Prep Time: 25 Minutes

Serves: 18

Ingredients:

- 1 Tbsp. of Vinegar, Apple Cider
- 1 Cup of Sugar, White
- 1 ½ Cups of Milk, Almond
- 2 tsp. of Baking Powder
- 1 ¼ tsp. of Vanilla Extract
- ½ tsp. of Baking Soda
- 2 Cups of Flour, All Purpose
- ½ tsp. of Salt
- ½ Cup of Coconut Oil, Warmed Up Until It Is A Liquid

Directions:

1. Preheat your oven to 350 degrees. While it heats up make sure to grease up to muffin pans with a generous amount of cooking spray or some muffin liners.
2. Using a large sized mixing bowl combine your dry ingredients and whisk together until mixed well. Using a separate mixing bowl combine all of your wet ingredients together and when you are ready pour into your dry ingredients. Stir until all of the ingredients are blended well together.
3. Spoon enough batter into your muffin pans so that each muffin tin is about ¾ full.
4. Place your muffin pans into your oven and bake for about 15 to 20 minutes or until the tops of the muffins spring back. Remove from oven and place on a cooling rack to cool off completely before your serve it.

Mouthwatering Tofu Pumpkin Pie

This recipe is a classic twist on your traditional pumpkin pie. Feel free to make this lighter in fat by using Splenda instead of half of your sugar.

Total Prep Time: 2 Hours

Serves: 6 to 8

Ingredients:
- ¾ Cup of Sugar, White
- 1, 10 Ounce Package of Tofu
- 1, 16 Ounce Can of Pumpkin, Puree
- ½ tsp. of Salt
- 1, 9 inch Pie Crust, Unbaked
- 1 tsp. of Cinnamon, Ground
- ¼ tsp. of Cloves, Ground
- ½ tsp. of Ginger, Ground

Directions:
1. Preheat your oven to 450 degrees.
2. While your oven heats up combine your pumpkin, cinnamon, tofu, ginger, salt and sugar together in a blender. Blend completely until the mixture reaches a smooth texture and make sure to pour into your piecrust.

3. Place your piecrust into your oven and bake for 15 minutes. Reduce your oven heat to 350 degrees and bake for an additional 40 minutes. Remove from oven and allow to cool completely before serving.

Vegan Style Brownies

I do not know who is not a fan of brownies. This recipe is not only Vegan friendly, but it is also great for those who suffer from dairy and egg allergies.

Total Prep Time: 50 Minutes

Serves: 6 to 8

Ingredients:
- 1 tsp. of Salt
- 2 Cups of Flour, All Purpose
- 1 tsp. of Baking Powder
- 1 Cup of Vegetable Oil
- 2 Cups of Sugar, White
- 1 Cup of Water
- ¾ Cup of Cocoa Powder, Unsweetened
- 1 tsp. of Vanilla Extract

Directions:
1. Preheat your oven to 350 degrees.
2. While your oven heats up use a large size mixing bowl and combine your cocoa powder, salt, flour, baking powder and sugar until all of the ingredients are mixed together. Pour this into your wet ingredients and stir until thoroughly combined.

3. Pour this into a baking pan and place into your oven to bake for the next 25 to 30 minutes or until the top of the brownies are no longer shiny. Remove from heat and allow brownies to cool for about 10 minutes before serving them.

Strawberries Mixed With Balsamic Vinegar

When you mix strawberries with some balsamic vinegar, you will help bring out the strawberries true flavor. Feel free to serve this dish with some pound cake or with some ice cream.

Total Prep Time: 1 Hour and 10 Minutes
Serves: 6
Ingredients:
- 16 Ounces of Strawberries, Fresh and Cut In Half
- 2 Tbsp. of Vinegar, Balsamic
- ¼ tsp of Black Pepper For Taste

- ¼ Cup of Sugar, White

Directions:
1. Place your strawberries into a bowl and drizzle some over the vinegar over it. Sprinkle with some sugar and stir as gently as you can to combine.
2. Grind some fresh pepper over it before serving.

Vegan Style Chocolate Pudding

This is one of the simplest recipes for dairy free chocolate pudding that you will ever find. You can use either ground cocoa or some ground chocolate to really bring out the flavor of this dessert dish.

Total Prep Time: 45 Minutes

Serves: 2

Ingredients:
- 3 Tbsp. of Cornstarch
- 1 ½ Cups of Milk, Soy
- ¼ Cup of Sugar, White
- ¼ Cup of Cocoa Powder, Unsweetened
- 2 Tbsp. of Water

- ¼ tsp. of Vanilla Extract

Directions:

1. In a small mixing bowl combine your water and cornstarch together until it begins to form a paste.
2. In a large sized saucepan over some medium heat combine your soymilk, cornstarch mix, sugar, ground cocoa and vanilla by stir them together. Cook and stir constantly until your pudding mixture begins to boil.
3. Remove from heat and allow the pudding to cool completely before placing it in your fridge to chill before serving.

Delicious Vegan Style Chocolate Cake

This is one of the simplest cakes that you can make. While it is very easy to make it is also surprisingly very tasty as well.

Total Prep Time: 60 Minutes

Serves: 4

Ingredients:

- 1/3 Cup of Vegetable Oil
- 1 ½ Cups of Flour, All Purpose
- ¼ Cup of Cocoa Powder
- 1 Cup of Sugar, White
- ½ tsp. of Salt
- 1 Cup of Water, Warm
- 1 tsp. of Vanilla Extract
- 1 tsp. of Baking Soda
- 1 tsp. of White Vinegar, Distilled

Directions:

1. Preheat your oven to 350 degrees. While your oven heats up grease a cake pan of your choice lightly with a generous amount of cooking spray.
2. In a medium sized mixing bowl combine your salt, flour, cocoa powder, sugar and baking soda. Add in the rest of your ingredients are stir thoroughly until the entire mixture is smooth.
3. Pour your cake batter into your cake pan and place into your oven. Bake your cake for 45 minutes. Remove from oven and allow to cool before serving.

Banana Flavored Cookies

Not only are these cookies incredibly nutritious, but they are extremely delicious as well.

Total Prep Time: 1 Hour and 10 Minutes
Serves: 8 to 10
Ingredients:
- 3 Bananas, Ripe and Mashed
- 1 Cup of Dates, Fresh, Pitted and Chopped Finely
- 1 tsp. of Vanilla Extract
- 2 Cups of Oats, Rolled
- 1/3 Cup of Vegetable Oil

Directions:
1. Preheat your oven to 350 degrees.
2. While your oven heats up use a large mixing bowl to mash your bananas. Then stir in your dates, vanilla extract, oats and oil. Mix well until all of the ingredients are thoroughly mixed and allow to sit for the next 15 minutes.
3. Drop a few spoonfuls of your batter onto a greased cookie sheet and place into your oven to bake for 20 minutes or until they cookies are golden brown in color. Remove from oven and allow to cool slightly before enjoying.

Basic Vanilla Cake

This dish is somewhat spongy and dense, making it a fairly simple cake recipe to make. Feel free to top if off with your favorite kind of vegan frosting.

Total Prep Time: 50 Minutes

Serves: 6 to 8

Ingredients:
- 1 Cup of Soymilk, Plain
- 1 tsp. of Baking Soda
- 1 Tbsp. of Vinegar, Apple Cider
- 1 Cup of Sugar, White
- 1 tsp. of Baking Powder
- 1 ½ Cups of Flour, All Purpose and Unbleached
- 1 tsp. of Baking Soda
- ¼ Cup of Water
- ½ tsp. of Salt
- ¼ tsp. of Extract, Almond
- 1/3 Cup of Canola Oil
- 1 Tbsp. of Vanilla Extract
- 1 Tbsp. of Lemon Juice, Fresh

Directions:

1. Preheat your oven to 350 degrees. While your oven heats up grease up a small to medium sized cake pan.
2. In a small to medium sized mixing bowl stir all of your ingredients together until you come up with a batter that is smooth and free of any lumps. Then pour your batter into your greased cake pan and place into your oven.
3. Bake your cake for 35 to 40 minutes and then remove from oven. Allow to cool slightly before removing it from the cake pan or adding some frosting to it.

Conclusion

Thank you again for downloading this cookbook!

Hopefully you have found some of the best vegan recipes that you will ever lay your eyes on. There are plenty of vegan breakfast, lunch, dinner and dessert recipes here that you can make to impress your friends or family.

I know that being on a Vegan diet can seem like a torture spell and a punishment for you, but that could not be any further from the truth. As long as you try your best to spice up your dish and remember to use as many fruits and veggies as possible, all of the dishes that you can make with the help of this cookbook will be the healthiest and most nutritious meals that you can possibly make.

Before you go, would you please do me a favor? As an Independent Author and Self-Publisher, I don't have a large publishing company promoting my books. What I do have though, are reviews from readers like you. In fact, reviews are the single most important way for me to be able to get in front of more readers. Without them, I have no chance in competing with the larger, more established authors.

Part 2

Sweet Potato Chickpea-less Hummus Vegan Bowl

Ingredients:

- To taste, high quality sea salt
- 3 small cloves of garlic that are minced
- ½ cup of fresh lemon juice
- 2 tablespoons of nutritional yeast
- ¾ cup of tahini
- 2 organic zucchinis that are peeled and chopped
- Chickpea-less Hummus
- Small amount of non-stick cooking spray
- To taste, high quality finely ground sea salt and black pepper
- 1 tablespoon of shelled hemp hearts, optional
- 1 cup of shredded kale; julienned
- 1 tablespoon + 1 teaspoon of virgin coconut oil that is unrefined

- 1 sweet potato that is scrubbed, peeled and cubed
- 1 ½ cups of vegetable broth
- ½ cup of uncooked quinoa that is rinsed

Directions:

1. Preheat oven at a temperature of 400°F.
2. In a small microwave safe dish, melt the 2 tablespoon coconut oil.
3. Before cutting it into cubes, scrub and peel the sweet potato first. When done, add in the sweet potato into an average sized mixing bowl and add in a tablespoon of melted coconut oil and salt, to taste.
4. Put the sweet potato on a foil covered baking sheet and let it bake atop the center rack for about 30 minutes, while flipping the potatoes occasionally every 10 minutes.
5. Get your Brussels sprouts and kale ready, and put in the mixture into the

bowl to coat in with the remainder of the coconut oil.

6. Add seasoning to it with the salt and pepper for taste and put on a different foil covered baking sheet.
7. Let it bake for 10 minutes while flipping it halfway through, once the potatoes are done.
8. Wash the quinoa until the water runs clear, in a mesh strainer.
9. Using a thin layer of a non-stick cooking spray, coat the bottom of an average size saucepan, and turn on the heat high. Add the washed quinoa and let it toast until the quinoa seems dry. There should be no water that will be visible.
10. Remain the burner on high, and add the 2 cups vegetable broth.
11. Boil the quinoa, cover it, and minimize the heat to low. Let it cook for 15 minutes.
12. Prepare your hummus while the quinoa is cooking.

13. Using a food processor, mix all the ingredients and blend it until the mixture turns completely smooth.
14. For assembling the bowl, fill in ¼ of the bowl with kale/Brussels sprout mixture, ¼ of the bowl with sweet potatoes, and finally half of the bowl with quinoa. Put a spoonful of the prepared hummus in the middle, and put on top of the hemp hearts and add pepper or salt if it is desired.

Quinoa Cauliflower with Almond Sauce Bowl

Ingredients:

- ½ teaspoon of sriracha
- ½ teaspoon of sesame oil
- ¼ teaspoon of salt
- 1 cup of water
- ½ cup of quinoa

- ¼ teaspoon of ginger powder
- 1 teaspoon of Sriracha, to taste
- 1 teaspoon of oil
- 1 teaspoon of sesame oil
- 1 small cauliflower that is chopped into small florets
- 2 tablespoons of water
- Large pinch of garlic powder and salt
- ½ teaspoon of oil
- 4-5 big collard greens leaves with its hard ribs removed and sliced chiffonade
- generous pinch of salt
- 3 tablespoons of coconut milk
- ½ teaspoon of sesame oil
- 2 teaspoons of extra virgin olive oil
- 2 teaspoons of maple syrup
- 1 teaspoon of apple cider vinegar
- 1-2 teaspoon of Sriracha, to taste
- ¼ teaspoon of garlic powder
- 2 teaspoons of ginger that is minced
- 3 tablespoons of Almond butter

Directions:

1. For the Quinoa, rinse the quinoa then cook it with the ½ teaspoon of sriracha, ½ teaspoon of sesame oil, ¼ teaspoon of salt, and 1 cup of water. Let it boil on average heat then let it cook at low medium heat covered partially for 10-15 minutes. Fluff it and keep it ready.

2. For the Roasted Cauliflower, in a bowl mix the 1 teaspoon sesame oil, 1 teaspoon oil, 1 teaspoon Sriracha, and ¼ teaspoon ginger powder. Toss in the Cauliflower. Sprinkle a little salt and let it bake at a preheated temperature of 425°F for 20-25 minutes.

3. For the Collard Greens, while the cauliflower is roasting, heat the oil in the pan on average heat. Add in the garlic, salt, and collard greens then let it cook for 1 minute. Add in the water, mix it, cover it, and let it cook on low medium heat until it turns lightly wilted.

4. For the Almond Sriracha Sauce, add the 3 tablespoons of almond butter, 2 teaspoon of minced ginger, ¼ teaspoon of garlic powder, 1-2 teaspoon of sriracha, 1 teaspoon of apple cider vinegar, 2 teaspoons of maple syrup, 2 teaspoons of extra virgin olive oil, ½ teaspoon of sesame oil, 3 tablespoons of coconut milk and a large pinch of salt in a blender. Blend it well and use. Taste and adjust the taste with salt and spice.

5. In a bowl, arrange everything and serve it with a considerable amount of drizzle of the dressing sesame seeds, and cilantro leaves.

Superfood Quinoa Bowl

Ingredients:

- Sriracha
- Walnut pesto and Spicy kale
- Hummus
- 2 tablespoons of silvered almonds
- 2 tablespoons of sesame seeds
- 2 tablespoons of flax seeds
- 2 cups of cooked quinoa
- 1 cup of shredded carrots
- 4 large beets that are peeled and cubed
- 1 bunch of asparagus

Directions:

1. Quinoa Preparation: In a pot on top of average heat, let 4 cups of water boil. Add in quinoa and a dash of sea salt and let it cook while it is covered until the moisture is absorbed for about 15 minutes. Take it off from the heat and keep the cover on.

2. In a saucepan, fill it with ½ inch with water and a dash of sea salt and let it boil. Cut off the white ends of the asparagus and add it into the boiling water, cover it, and let it cook for 2 minutes or just until it turns soft but remains firm. Drain the water and wash it with cold water to halt the cooking process. Cut it into 1 inch sections.
3. For the assembly, put in the quinoa with almonds, sesame seeds, and flax seeds. Layer all the vegetables in a big bowl and dress it with sriracha, hummus and pesto.

Burrito-Added Cauliflower Rice Bowl

Ingredients:

- To taste, salt and pepper
- 2 tablespoons of olive oil
- 1 small head of raw cauliflower of any color that is cut into medium florets
- fresh Cilantro leaves
- Fried corn tortilla chips, fresh
- Jalapeños that are pickled
- 1 ripe avocado that is sliced or cut into chunks
- 2 small handfuls of shredded cheddar cheese

- 2 spoonfuls of spicy salsa
- 2 cups of kale or spinach that are floppy and sautéed in olive oil and garlic
- 1 cup of black beans that are warmed
- 2 big portions of cauliflower rice

Directions:

1. For the cauliflower rice, put the florets in the food processor fitted with the blade attachment. Let it process until the cauliflower is grounded into fine bits.
2. Put a big skillet on top of average heat. Add in the olive oil. Add in the cauliflower bits to the heated pan and toss it to combine. Let it cook until the cauliflower rice has browned and softened slightly, for about 6-8 minutes. Season it generously with the pepper and salt. Add in any different seasoning you might want. Take it out from the heat and spoon it into two big bowls. If there is any excess rice, refrigerate it for up to 5 days.
3. For the burrito bowl, start making it with a big shallow bowl. Spoon the cauliflower rice onto the plate. Next to the rice, spoon the warmed black beans. Next to the beans, spoon the sautéed kale. Top it generously with fresh cilantro leaves, fried tortilla chips, pickled jalapeños, ripe avocado,

shredded cheese, and hot salsa. Enjoy it!

Marinated Tofu Brown Rice Bowl

Ingredients:

- 1 cup of cabbage kimchi
- 3 cups of cooked brown rice
- 1 big red bell pepper that is sliced
- 3 tablespoons of grape seed oil or sunflower oil
- 1 tablespoon of dark sesame oil
- 2 tablespoons of mirin
- 2 tablespoons of light miso
- 2 teaspoons of lime juice
- 1 tablespoon of honey or agave nectar
- ⅛ teaspoon of cayenne, optional
- 1 clove of garlic that is minced
- 1 tablespoon of ginger that is minced
- 3 tablespoons of soy sauce
- One 14 ounce block of organic extra-firm tofu that is cut into 8 slices

Directions:

1. Preheat oven at a temperature of 375°F. Line the sheet pan using parchment. Pat-dry each of the slices of tofu using paper towels.
2. Whisk together the oils, mirin, miso, lime juice, honey or agave nectar, cayenne, garlic, ginger, and soy sauce. Put it into a dish large enough to accommodate all of the tofu slices in one layer. Put the tofu slices in the marinade and turn it over. Let it marinate for 15 minutes, while turning it once or twice. Put it to the baking sheet. Add in the peppers to the dish with marinade and toss it to coat thoroughly, and then put it on the baking sheet in one layer.
3. Put the baking sheet inside the oven and let it roast for 15-20 minutes, while turning the peppers once using the tongs, just until the edges of the tofu begins to color and the marinade begins to set on the surface, and the peppers begin to sizzle and color on the edges. Take it out from the heat.

4. If it is desired, heat the kimchi in a small pan. Spoon the rice into the 4 wide bowls. Top it with peppers, tofu and kimchi. If wanted, douse the rice with the remainder of the marinade from the tofu, and then serve.

Chickpeas and Roasted Cauliflower Bowl with Lemon-Dijon Dressing

Ingredients:

- 2 tablespoons of grape seed oil
- To taste, salt and pepper
- ⅛ teaspoon of crushed red pepper flakes
- 1 bunch (small) of flat leaf parsley that is diced
- 1 cup of dry quinoa
- 1 can of chickpeas that is rinsed
- 1 head of cauliflower that is cut into florets
- ⅛ teaspoon of fine sea salt
- ¼ cup of extra virgin coconut oil
- 1-2 teaspoons of Dijon style mustard
- 1 ½ tablespoons of fresh lemon juice

Directions:

1. Preheat oven at a temperature of 400°F.
2. In a big bowl, toss in the chickpeas and cauliflower with oil. Sprinkle the salt, red pepper flakes, and pepper. Equally speared on a previously prepared baking sheet and let it roast in the oven for about 20-35 minutes while tossing the mixture halfway.
3. While the vegetables are cooking, prepare the quinoa. Mix 2 cups of water and 1 cup of quinoa. Let it boil. Minimize the heat to low, cover it and let it cook until the quinoa has already absorbed the liquid that it can be easily fluffed using a fork, for about 15 minutes.
4. Prepare dressing by mixing the ⅛ teaspoon of fine grained sea salt, ¼ cup of extra virgin olive oil, 1-2 teaspoon of Dijon-style mustard, and 1 ½ tablespoons of fresh lemon juice and whisking it until it turns smooth.
5. Mix the chickpeas and cauliflower with the quinoa. Drizzle it with the dressing and put the minced parsley on top.

Falafel Roasted Chickpeas Entree

Ingredients:

- Spicy sauce
- Tahini Sauce
- Hummus
- Turnip or cabbage that is pickled
- Sliced tomatoes
- Sliced cucumber
- Shredded lettuce
- Tabbouleh
- Falafel Roasted Chickpeas
- 2 tablespoons of fresh parsley
- A pinch of cardamom
- A pinch of cayenne
- ¼ teaspoon of black pepper
- 1 teaspoon of kosher salt
- 1 teaspoon of coriander
- 1 ½ teaspoons of cumin
- 3 cloves of garlic that are minced
- ½ cup of red onion that is chopped
- 1 tablespoon of lemon juice
- 2 tablespoons of olive oil
- 3 cups of chickpeas

- 2 teaspoons of fresh parsley, optional
- A pinch of cayenne
- ¼ teaspoon of salt
- 1 tablespoon of olive oil

- 3-5 tablespoons of water
- 1-3 cloves of garlic that are minced
- 3 tablespoons of lemon juice
- ⅓ cup of tahini

Directions:

1. Bowl assembly instructions: Add in some of the tabbouleh, and then next to the tabbouleh add in a handful of lettuce that is previously shredded, next is the chickpeas, then some cucumber, tomato, dollop of hummus and pickled turnip. Drizzle tahini sauce in the bowl. Add hot sauce if needed.
2. Falafel Roasted Chickpeas instructions: Preheat oven at a temperature of 375°F and line the baking sheet using a parchment paper.
3. Wash and drain the chickpeas then put them in a big bowl

4. Add in the cardamom, cayenne, pepper, salt, coriander, cumin, garlic, onion, lemon juice, and olive oil in the bowl and toss it until the chickpeas are equally coated.
5. Put the chickpeas onto the previously prepared baking sheet and spread it out into a single even layer.
6. Let it bake for 35-40 minutes while stirring it one time halfway.
7. Let it cool slightly and put the fresh parsley.
8. Tahini sauce instruction: In a small bowl, whisk together the salt, olive oil, 3 tablespoons of water, garlic, and lemon juice until it turns smooth. Add in more water to be able to get to the desired consistency. Stir in the parsley.

Cranberry Vegan Salad Sandwich

Ingredients:

- ½ teaspoon each of mineral salt and freshly ground pepper, to taste
- ½ cup of scallions with thinly sliced, white and green parts
- ½ cup of walnuts or pecans that are roughly chopped
- ½ cup of organic dried cranberries that chopped fresh
- 1 cup of celery that is diced
- 3 cups of cooked chickpeas that are drained and washed

Directions:

1. Begin by mixing the dressing. In a small bowl, mix the tahini, maple syrup, vinegar, and water. Leave it aside so the flavors mix together. This can be prepared ahead a day or two

refrigerated until it is ready to be used. Add an additional tad of water or vinegar, to thin out the dressing, as desired. If vegan mayo is used, add 2 additional tablespoons.
2. Using a medium or large bowl, add the chickpeas and mash it roughly using a strong fork or potato crusher. Add in the pepper, salt, scallions, nuts, cranberries, celery and dressing. Mix well. Serve it in room temperature or refrigerate it to chill for an hour before serving it.
3. Serve it with your favorite bread as either open or closed face sandwich, or on top of leafy veggies. You may serve and enjoy the salad as it is.

Roasty Soba Entrée

Ingredients:

- Several dashes of fresh black pepper
- ¼ teaspoon of salt
- 1 tablespoon of olive oil
- 1 medium head cauliflower that is cut into big florets
- 2 cups of cooked brown or green lentils
- 8 ounces of buckwheat soba noodles
- Fresh herbs, optional

Directions:

1. Cook first the lentils if your lentils aren't the prepared ones. Preheat oven at a temperature of 425°F and chop cauliflower into big florets while water for the soba is going to a boil. An easier way to do it by chopping them into half lengthwise, while peeling off the leafy base, and then pulling off the florets using your hands.

2. When the water boils, make a prepared soba using the instructions written in the package. Once it is already cooked, drain it, and leave it aside, while rinsing it with cold water just to prevent it from sticking.
3. Using a parchment paper, line a big rimmed baking sheet and spray using a non-stick cooking spray. Toss in the cauliflower with the pepper, salt, and olive oil. Let it roast for 20 minutes, while flipping it once, just until the aromatic is nicely toasted.
4. For the meantime, put in the ¼ cup of mellow white miso, ¼ cup of tahini, 1 clove of garlic, and ½ - ¾ cup of water in a small blender. Begin with ½ cup of water, then add ¼ more to make thin, if you desire.
5. To assemble the bowls, divide the soba noodles in large bowls. Top it with cauliflower, lentils and a considerable amount of sauce. Garnish it with herbs and then serve it.

Peas Shallots Burmese Fried Rice

Ingredients:

- Cilantro leaves, fresh
- Lime wedges
- 1 cup of frozen green peas
- Optional, hot sauce
- Optional, fried shallots
- 1 teaspoon of salt, gluten-free soy sauce or fish sauce
- 4 cups of cold cooked brown rice
- ½ cup of thinly sliced shallots
- ¼ teaspoon of turmeric
- 1 ½ tablespoons of olive oil

Directions:

1. Over medium high heat, heat the wok. Add in the oil, and then add the shallots and turmeric. Have it sautéed until the shallots turn translucent for about 3-4 minutes. Add in the cooked rice, and use hands to break the chunks up. Add in the peas and salt,

and toss it well, while cooking until the rice is well heated and the peas are already just cooked.
2. Serve it with browned shallots, cooked beans, and hot sauce, cilantro, and wedges of lime.

Cauliflower with Orange Sauce Entrée

Ingredients:

- 1 small head cauliflower that is cut into small florets
- 1 teaspoon of oil
- ¼ cup of gluten-free flour
- ⅓ cup of corn starch
- ⅓ cup of water
- 1 tablespoon of flaxseed meal & 2 tablespoon of water that is allowed to sit until it has thicken
- 6 thinly sliced green onions
- 3-4 cloves of garlic that are peeled and zested
- 2 tablespoons of oil
- 1 teaspoon of brown sugar
- 1 teaspoon of corn starch
- ¼ cup of orange juice
- 2 tablespoons of rice wine vinegar
- 2 tablespoons of gluten-free soy sauce
- A zest of 1 orange & juice of orange
- 1 teaspoon of oil

Directions:

1. Whisk together the 1 teaspoon of oil, ¼ cup of corn starch, ⅓ cup of water, 1 tablespoon of flaxseed meal mix until a nice batter is formed. Remember that it should not be too thick.
2. Heat the skillet with ½ cup of oil on medium or high heat. Make it a point to check if it is already properly heated.
3. Dip the small floret into the batter one at a time until it is covered. Fry it in oil until it turns completely brown and let it drain on a paper towel lined on top of the plate.
4. Using another skillet or cleaned skillet, heat the garlic and oil for a minute. Add in the juice, zest, and green onions. Cook for 1 minute more. Add in the vinegar and soy sauce, and then let it boil. Put in the cauliflower into the skillet then allow it coat thoroughly.
5. Place it on a scoop of rice.

6. Using the same skillet put in the remaining ingredients for the orange sauce and let it boil for 1 minute while stirring it constantly. Drizzle over the rice and orange cauliflower.

About the Author

Daryl Morris is author of several cookbooks on Vegan diet. He has written research papers on the topic and currently lives in California.

www.ingramcontent.com/pod-product-compliance
Lightning Source LLC
LaVergne TN
LVHW012000070526
838202LV00054B/4983